Love at Turtle Beach

Romances for Seniors

seniorality

Love at Turtle Beach -
Jamie Stonebridge, Chrissie Stephen

Copyright © 2024
Seniorality / Everbreeze Media Oy

This is a work of fiction. Names and characters are the product of the author's imagination and any resemblance to actual persons, living or dead, is entirely coincidental.

Set in 22 pt EB Garamond

Chapter 1
The Turtle Adventure Begins

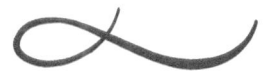

THE WEATHERED old green Land Rover bounced along the dusty track. Claire looked out the back of the canvas soft top to watch the billowing clouds of sand it churned up. The landscape appeared barren, dotted only with gorse bushes and inland cliffs carved by the sea millions of years before. Nicos, the driver, regularly shouted back to Claire to ensure she and Kurt were fine in the back. Next to the driver sat another passenger, named Johann.

Twenty minutes later, Claire and the other two new arrivals stood atop the sand dunes. Below them sprawled a vast, curved sandy beach, fringed by the twinkling azure waters of the Mediterranean.

The beach was stunningly beautiful and was going to be 'home' for all of them for the next eight weeks.

The four of them walked down the makeshift wooden staircase surrounded by thorny bushes. The three new arrivals each carrying a laden rucksack. At the bottom of the steps there was a small wooden hut. In front of it, a long table and two benches were arranged under a large shady canopy.

Nicos officially welcomed them, "Kalosorisate steen Kypro - welcome to Cyprus - and to the Lara Turtle Project, which we have been successfully running for 50 years. My name is Nicos Paphitis, and I work for the Fisheries Department, overseeing the project. Thank you for volunteering to help us here at the turtle station. I hope you have a really good time here. It's hard work, but we will have time to relax too."

He then asked the three new arrivals to introduce themselves. Johann was from Salzburg, Austria, studying to be a veterinarian. Kurt's home was just outside Munich, where he was studying Nature Conservation and Landscape Planning. Claire introduced herself, explaining that she was in her second year studying marine biology at the University of Southampton in England, and her family was living in Amsterdam, where her father managed a large pharmaceutical company.

A short distance away, there were two large faded cream-colored frame tents that made Claire smile as she looked at them and wondered if they could actually be older than her grandmother!

"Right, let's get you settled into your tents," said Nicos enthusiastically.

Nicos showed the two young men to the first tent and Claire to the second tent. Inside the tent, Claire found two camp beds just inside the flap, both strewn with duvets and personal belongings. On the far side, a third camp bed stood completely bare. Claire put her rucksack next to it and took the chance to swap her trainers for flip flops and apply some more sunscreen.

By the time she had re-emerged from the tent, everyone else had gathered under the canopy. Shortly afterwards, the kettle could be heard whistling, and Nicos made everyone a mug of tea.

"You may think this is a very strange choice of drink in such warm weather, but in India, the British always drank tea in hot weather, and it does seem to quench the thirst," Nicos explained.

The group happily chatted together. Claire found herself repeatedly drawn to look at the view, which really was so beautiful. There were just a handful of people on the beach, all of whom repeatedly popped down to the sea for a cooling dip.

At the back of the beach, there were a series of information boards on wooden posts, standing some distance behind two rows of large, round metal cages that resembled lobster pots. Nicos encouraged everyone to finish their drinks so that he could quickly show them around. He kept apologizing for his 'terrible English,' although to Claire, it sounded perfect.

Although he had been born in Paphos, the nearest town to the turtle project, Nicos had attended the English School in Nicosia. This school had long been regarded as the top school in Cyprus. All the lessons were taught in English, but the students also studied Modern Greek, making them totally bilingual.

Nicos showed the three arrivals where the washing-up facilities were and the makeshift shower made from a hose pipe attached to a tall, vertical wooden post. There was also a small camping toilet cubicle. Water had to be treated like liquid gold as it came from a small water tank at the top of the dunes, which was hard work and time-consuming to refill.

They were examining the information boards when Nicos waved to three people who had suddenly appeared on the beach, each carrying a bag of shopping. Everyone gathered around the table as Nicos introduced the 'happy shoppers.' There were two young women, Juliette from Paris, and Maria, who was Cypriot. The third person was a tall Danish man with wavy blonde hair named Nils. All of them had volunteered to work at the seasonal turtle station too.

As Nicos had explained just before the group's arrival, the aim of the project was to protect the turtle hatchlings (baby turtles). He had described how two species of marine turtles come ashore on several beaches in Cyprus: the Loggerhead (*Caretta caretta*) and the Green (*Chelonia midas*). Both species were endangered, and the future of the Green Turtle was now hanging in the balance.

He also explained that although females can lay more than 100 eggs every two weeks during the breeding season, in reality, only one in 100 of these hatchlings would make it to adulthood. The group spent the final hours of daylight preparing for the night ahead when they would be working. They placed their night clothes and bottles of water carefully on their camp beds where they could easily find them in darkness.

Claire volunteered to join the group that was walking along the beach to request all the holidaymakers to leave as it was now an hour before sunset. The rest of the group went to the beaches on either side of Lara to do the same. As the final family left the beach, Nils, Juliette, and Claire once again walked the length of the beach, this time carefully checking that no litter had been left as this would injure the female marine turtles when they came ashore to lay their eggs.

Claire found herself alone on the beach as the sun began to sink in the sky. She stared in awe at its beauty and did not move until the sun had sunk below the horizon. Nicos had told them all that there is no dusk in Cyprus, and he had certainly not exaggerated - sunset turned to night incredibly quickly.

Claire found herself wondering about what the next few weeks would bring. She had applied to join the Lara Turtle Project as a volunteer as she had no other plans for the summer and had just broken up with her boyfriend at Uni, which was definitely the right decision.

Nevertheless, Claire found herself missing his companionship. She looked up at the inky sky and remembered that they had been told earlier that they would get an amazing view of the stars and planets as there was no light pollution.

Nicos had told them that the use of torches and the lantern in the hut must be kept to a minimum as turtles can easily get disoriented by lights as they navigate by moonlight and the earth's magnetic fields. Shortly afterwards, they all gathered around the large wooden table for a simple meal of pasta tossed in olive oil, with salad and village bread -

which Kurt had prepared. They ate by the light of two tiny candles.

They took turns patrolling the beaches in pairs. Nikos took a couple of volunteers each time to check the first and third beaches, using the Land Rover on the sandy track as the tide was in, making it impossible to scramble over the rocks.

Claire had been paired with Maria, who had started work at Lara three weeks earlier. They walked silently side by side, carefully scanning the beach, looking for any movement and listening for the sound of flicking sand, which would indicate that a female turtle was covering the chamber she had dug in the sand and filled with her eggs. Depending on their species and age, female turtles usually lay between 80-150 eggs.

When they reached the far end of the beach, Maria suggested that they sit on the rocks for a few minutes to enjoy the lulling sound of the waves and the shimmer of the moonlight on them. The pair sat on the rocks, and Maria sighed, "It is beautiful here, isn't it? I live in Nicosia, and because it is inland and well away from any cooling breeze, it gets incredibly hot in the summer – often 104 F in August."

They continued chatting as they got up to walk back to the hut. Maria asked Claire about the marine biology course, what it was like in Amsterdam, and whether she had a boyfriend. Claire explained that she had recently ended things with her boyfriend at university because she found him too self-centered and controlling. She asked Maria the same question.

"There have been several attractive men at my university that I have liked, but in Cyprus, there are still difficulties in going out with someone. Your parents ask you a million questions, and even if it is just your second date, they are considering whether he is good husband material! I suppose this is because things have changed so much here. My parents married 30 years ago in an arranged marriage. My mother's parents knew my father's parents, and they all decided that they would make a good couple."

"Wow!" gasped Claire, "Imagine that! What happens if you don't like the man your parents have chosen? I have decided that coming to Cyprus is the change I needed. I am looking forward to making some great new friends like you, but I am not rushing into another romance."

Maria laughed and grabbed Claire's arm, "I think that we are going to be very good friends, and we can enjoy our time at Lara without love getting in the way!"

Chapter 2
A Break from Routine

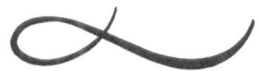

ALEKOS walked out of the operating theater and carefully removed his mask and gown, pleased with how the four-hour operation had gone. He meticulously washed his hands and arms and spun around when he heard Pavlos, the top surgeon, and four nurses pushing the swing door and entering the room.

"Thank you very much for all your help in there," said Pavlos, smiling as he removed his mask. "You should be really proud of what we have achieved this afternoon. Our young motorcyclist will certainly thank us in years to come; his spinal injuries were worse than I first suspected. Alekos, you did really well. I admit that I took a back seat and let you do all the hard work now that you are in the final year of your residency and have gained such a wealth of experience."

Everyone wished the popular surgeon a good evening. The nurses also congratulated Alekos and commented on how skillful he had been. One of the nurses quipped, "You have obviously impressed the boss, which is brilliant. I know he has already recommended that you stay on here at Nicosia General."

Soon, Alekos was on his way home. He thoroughly enjoyed the 15-minute walk to his apartment as it gave him time to unwind. Long operations were always incredibly tiring as they demanded his utmost concentration. As he walked, he felt the change in him, which he described as 'rejoining the normal world.'

Alekos had wanted to be a neurosurgeon since he was a boy. He had grown up in a medical family; his father was a highly respected orthopedic surgeon, and his uncle was a neurosurgeon. Throughout his schooldays, he had loved all the science subjects and had excelled in all his examinations. He was particularly fascinated by the human brain, and at 16 years old, he had decided that neurosurgery was the career path for him. He applied to study at The National University of Athens and was delighted when the letter arrived confirming that he had a place.

Alekos enjoyed his years of study, but nevertheless, he could not wait to put all he had learned into practice and was delighted when he had been offered the chance to do his residency in Nicosia working alongside Pavlos. During the six years he had spent in Athens, he had always looked forward to returning home to Cyprus for the holidays. It was great to see his parents and wider family and to catch up with some of his school friends.

His closest friend for the whole time he was at the school was Nicos Paphitis. Nicos had been a fun-loving boy who was determined to be a marine biologist. As his family home was in Paphos, Nicos had spent the weeks with his Yaya (Grandmother) who lived close to the school in Nicosia.

As he walked along the streets towards his apartment, Alekos vividly recalled the many afternoons and evenings he had spent with Nicos at his grandmother's house. He laughed when he remembered how the pair of them would sit at the huge kitchen table with their study books all around them, and Yaya would supply them with endless things to eat and drink.

In no time at all, Alekos had reached his apartment, tapped his code onto the pad by the main door, and was turning the key in the lock of his own front door.

Alekos sat and read for a while before preparing himself dinner. He hated eating alone, but there was a limit to the number of meals he could eat in the hospital canteen, and at the end of a busy day, there was often too much noise. He thought about the weekend ahead. He had planned on seeing his parents, but his mom had telephoned early that morning and reminded him that they were off to the Troodos mountains to see friends.

Alekos looked at his empty plate and smiled as an idea came into his mind. Would it be possible to travel to Paphos and spend the weekend helping Nicos and his turtle team? It would be a great chance to have some colorful discussions with Nicos and to walk the beaches in the early hours looking for marine turtles. Alekos usually managed to squeeze in at least one trip to the turtle station each summer, and thinking about it, he suddenly felt that he could do with a break from hospital life.

He tried calling Nicos but couldn't reach him. He remembered that there was no cell phone coverage on the beach, and the only time you could get through was when Nicos was on the top of the dunes or, better still, in town.

Having decided on his weekend plans, Alekos couldn't settle and found himself repeatedly trying to call Nicos. Eventually, he was successful.

"Hi Alekos, how are you doing?" Alekos was delighted to hear his friend's voice. They chatted briefly, and Nicos sounded delighted that his friend would be spending the weekend with him.

"It will be cozy in the tent as there are three of us in it already! Don't forget to bring your camp bed! Can you persuade your mom to make some of her wonderful fasoulia (haricot beans with mixed vegetables) and a tray of her heavenly pastries? As you know, the cooking facilities are very limited."

They said their goodbyes, and Alekos mentioned that he wouldn't get away early from work on Friday, so he would leave early on Saturday morning to make the three-hour trip. Alekos lifted his rucksack down from the top of the cupboard in the spare bedroom and quickly gathered his shorts, T-shirts, and swimming trunks, popping them into his sack. Having made the decision to head to Lara, he already felt better.

Friday was usually a quieter day at the hospital, and Alekos was relieved because it had been necessary to rearrange his operating schedule as the young motorcyclist had been admitted the previous day as an emergency. Once work was over, Alekos walked through the staff car park. He had purposely driven his car to the hospital because he was visiting his parents straight afterward to collect the food order for Nicos!

He rang the doorbell, and within moments he was being tightly embraced by his mom! In an instant, he felt like he was five years old, but it was still a comforting feeling, just as it had always been. A short while later, his father arrived home, muttering about the number of rugby players regularly in need of an orthopedic surgeon! They enjoyed a delicious meal together, and not for the first time, Alekos told his mom how much he missed her cooking.

As Alekos was planning an early start the next morning, he did not stay late, even though he enjoyed seeing his parents, and he knew they wanted an early start for the journey to the mountains. He followed his mom into the kitchen where two large plastic containers stood on the table waiting for him. He gave his mom a big hug and thanked her for all the cooking. She smiled as she teased him, "Well, I think it's time both you and Nicos found yourselves wives that are good cooks."

Chapter 3
Beach Life

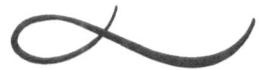

ALEKOS stood at the top of the sand dunes and looked down on the beautiful sandy beach below and the sea stretching as far as the horizon. He bounded down the broad wooden steps like an excited child and grinned as he saw his friend standing at the bottom on the sand watching him.

"Kalimera filos mou – Good morning, my friend," he greeted Nicos eagerly, who grabbed the large tubs of food that Alekos was carrying and put them safely in the hut. He then climbed back up the wooden steps with his friend to help carry the camp bed, leaving Alekos to manage his pack. The two then sat down outside under the canopy outside the hut and enjoyed a small cup of thick Cyprus coffee accompanied by a chilled glass of water.

Nicos explained that most of the volunteers were still asleep as it had been a busy night with three turtles coming ashore – two on the main beach and one on Lara One. The men went and checked that all was good with the new nests that the team had carefully moved from where they were laid and relocated to the Turtle Station where they were protected by the special metal cages. Many years before, the team had missed a turtle coming ashore and, to their horror, had woken the following morning to see a fox digging up the nest and eating the precious eggs – lesson learned.

Alekos spent much of the morning working with Nicos on strengthening the wooden staircase as some of the wood had started to move under the sheer weight of sand. Alekos and Nicos were struggling with getting the top wooden step perfectly in place when a young woman with long brown hair tied in a loose bun came springing up the steps.

When she reached their level, Nicos introduced her to Alekos. Claire smiled shyly and shook Alekos' hand, saying "Kalimera – good morning, I'm afraid this is the only Greek word I know, Maria has promised to teach me more!" Alekos observed her closely as she discussed with Nicos about the dwindling water supply in the tank. He noticed her dark brown inquisitive eyes and kind demeanor. Momentarily distracted, he heard Nicos telling her that he and Alekos would fetch some water supplies after lunch. Claire skipped back down the wooden steps as Alekos watched her, a detail not missed by his friend. They continued their work before heading back down to the hut.

The table was set for everyone, with Maria having prepared a huge Greek salad, thick slices of bread, creamy cucumber and yogurt tzatziki, and chickpea hummus. Nicos introduced each volunteer to Alekos, joking about their long-standing friendship despite supporting different football teams since they were 12 years old. They discussed the project's success from the previous night and were briefly approached by a holidaymaker whose daughter wanted to see a turtle. Nicos explained gently that it wouldn't be possible.

After the father and daughter left, Nicos outlined the plans for the afternoon. Many volunteers were exhausted, so he suggested that he and Alekos could go for water while Maria and Claire rested in the shade to attend to any inquiries from holidaymakers. "The rest of you can have a well-earned siesta – afternoon naps," Nicos declared. He mentioned the upcoming Full Moon, often referred to as a 'Turtle Moon' due to turtles favoring it for egg-laying, implying they might be busy again that night.

The afternoon passed swiftly as Nicos and Alekos loaded the large water canister into the back of the Land Rover and headed to the next village to fill it.

Upon their return, they faced the laborious task of siphoning water into the tank. It was hot work, and they were grateful to retreat under the canopy. As soon as they arrived at the hut, Claire reappeared with two bottles of cool water, which Nicos and Alekos gratefully drank.

Most of the other volunteers were still lounging on their beds, while Nils could be spotted at the far end of the beach, navigating over the rocks after his walk to check the next beach. Nicos gathered everyone and announced it was time for an activity. He shared the local legend surrounding a rock protruding from the water about 200 feet from the shore, believed to bestow eternal youth to anyone swimming around it three times clockwise. Excitedly, they all dashed into the sea, laughing and racing to reach the rock. Nils, with his long legs, surged ahead, while Maria and Claire opted for a more leisurely swim together around the rock. Alekos, not far behind, teased them about how they would prove their eternal youth to each other.

Upon returning to shore, they joked about forgetting their shoes, feeling the uncomfortable heat of the sand beneath their feet. Shortly after, they commenced their evening routine of urging holidaymakers to leave the beach and meticulously inspecting all three beaches for any harmful debris. As Claire meticulously checked the area around the turtle cages and information boards, she paused to admire the photographs, especially those of the baby turtles making their way to the sea. She eagerly anticipated witnessing this firsthand, knowing she'd have to wait about six weeks for the incubation period to conclude.

Suddenly, she felt a presence and turned to find Alekos nearby, also studying the photographs. "I can't describe how incredible it is to witness the young turtles emerge from their nest in the sand," he remarked. "Despite their small size, they make their way to the sea remarkably quickly." Claire smiled, expressing her eagerness to witness it herself. "Are there ever any issues preventing the baby turtles from successfully leaving the nest?" she inquired.

"Each nest is carefully checked to ensure it's empty," Alekos explained gently. "Most hatchlings emerge within a few hours, but sometimes they get too tired or struggle to break out of their shells. To check the nest, you have to gently dig down with your fingers. The nest is round, about eight inches wide, and can be up to 30 inches deep. When the eggs are first laid, the nest resembles a collection of white ping-pong balls."

Alekos smiled as he reached out to point at a photograph on the board. Claire noticed his pale complexion and long fingers, leading her to speculate that he likely worked indoors, possibly as a musician. Alekos's gentle voice brought her back to reality as he spoke about the delicate hatchlings. "Sometimes, you'll find a small, weak hatchling that needs to be gently removed and kept in that large shaded tank over there for a day or so to ensure they're ready for their journey to freedom," he explained.

Their conversation was interrupted by the sound of footsteps on the sand, and Maria appeared, announcing that dinner was ready and smelled delicious.

Over the meal, Nicos organized the night shift teams. Since Claire and Maria had done the 02:00 shift the previous night, they were granted a decent night's sleep and assigned to walk the beaches at midnight and 06:00. Meanwhile, others would take shifts throughout the night to monitor for turtles.

Just before midnight, Maria gently patted Claire awake, and they strolled along the moonlit beach, hoping to spot a turtle but finding none. Disappointed, they returned to their tent, where Claire struggled to sleep and eventually decided to sit outside, captivated by the moonlit scenery.

"Kalispera – Good evening – may I join you?" Claire recognized Alekos's voice, which inexplicably made her heart race. They sat together in silence for a while before Alekos inquired about her university course and future plans. Claire shared a bit about herself, admitting she only knew Alekos from his time at the English School with Nicos.

Alekos chuckled, describing his work at the hospital in Nicosia and his upcoming role as a surgeon. As they chatted, Maria and Nils returned, surprised to find them awake at such an hour. Claire and Alekos explained they couldn't sleep, then continued their conversation, comparing their families and lifestyles.

After a few minutes of silence, Alekos gently suggested they walk along the water's edge. Claire agreed, and as she rose, Alekos reached out his hand, which she found strong and reassuring. They walked hand in hand along the beach, eventually settling on the rocks at the far end.

'Claire, I know we've only just met this morning, but I already feel that you're someone very special, someone I'd really like to get to know more,' Alekos expressed as he rose from the rock, extending his hand to Claire once again. She accepted it, and he drew her close, planting gentle kisses on her cheeks. 'I think I shall call you my English Rose,' he added with a laugh.

Walking hand in hand along the beach, Alekos suddenly stopped and gazed at Claire tenderly. 'I don't know how to say this, but sadly, I must head back to Nicosia early tomorrow evening. It's a three-hour drive, and I need to prepare for a busy Monday at the hospital,' he explained, pulling her close once more and showering her cheeks with more kisses. 'For the first time, Claire, I'm not looking forward to going to work!' he confessed with a chuckle. 'But I think it would be lovely to return here next weekend.'

Claire smiled warmly at Alekos. 'I think that would be really lovely, and I would like that very much. I'm sad that time is flying by, but I fully understand your work commitments. What you do to help so many people is truly amazing,' she said sincerely.

As they arrived at the hut, Alekos and Claire paused to bid each other goodnight. Alekos kissed Claire gently on her lips and whispered, 'Kalinichta – goodnight, my English rose.' Claire retreated to her tent, her heart pounding with a mix of emotions. She questioned herself about the rapidity of her feelings for Alekos and the potential complications they might bring.

However, before she could find any answers, sleep overtook her, and she drifted off into a peaceful slumber.

Although Claire was enjoying a peaceful slumber, it was short-lived. Just after seven in the morning, Juliette, Kurt, and Nils were buzzing with excitement, rousing everyone from their sleep.

"Claire, Maria, you have to get up! There are three new turtle nests on this beach and another on Lara One—it's amazing!" Juliette exclaimed. "It's true what they say about the Turtle Moon! Nils and I saw two of the turtles digging their nests, and Nicos and Alekos saw the third turtle on Lara One just heading for the sea."

Realizing there was no chance of sleeping in, Claire quickly dressed and headed outside, carrying her wash bag to the sink. After brushing her teeth, she was returning to her tent when Alekos emerged from inside the hut.

"Kalimera—Good morning, my English rose, would you like coffee?" he greeted her.

"Oh yes, please," Claire replied. She entered the tent, tossed her wash bag on her camp bed, and joined Alekos at the table in front of the hut.

"Kalimera agapi mou—Good morning my love," Alekos said affectionately. "Did you hear about all our excitement? I'm not surprised to see a few turtles coming ashore because the Turtle Moon is very special for us, and so..."

He leaned forward, gently taking Claire's hand from the table and kissing it. "You know we all have plenty of work to do now?" he continued. He disappeared into the hut and returned with a Cyprus coffee for Claire, just as everyone gathered around the table.

Nicos quickly explained the process for handling the new turtle nests, emphasizing the importance of carefully digging them up and transporting them to the hatchery. Alekos reminded his friend to mention measuring the depth of the original turtle nest. Nicos grinned and thanked him, acknowledging Alekos's vital point.

"Yes, Alekos makes a very important point," Nicos agreed. "It's essential to measure the depth of the sand above the first layer of eggs and the total depth of the nest. Scientists have established that the temperature of the nest during the incubation period determines the sex of the hatchlings, so we must try to replicate this."

Alekos volunteered to take the Land Rover over to the beach at Lara One and asked if he had a volunteer to help him.

Claire didn't hesitate and offered to assist. As they headed for the wooden steps to climb the sand dune, Nicos gave his friend a knowing grin.

Upon arrival at Lara One, Alekos mentioned to Claire that they needed to work quickly as the sun was already heating up. They worked seamlessly together, with Alekos occasionally brushing Claire's fingers with his own.

Once they safely secured the precious turtle eggs in the insulated box, Alekos carefully carried it back to the Land Rover. Then, with a swift motion, he swept Claire into his arms, softly kissing her and expressing gratitude for making his weekend so special. He admitted he already knew he would miss her greatly when he returned to Nicosia.

As they made their way back to the Turtle station, Alekos asked Claire if it would be alright to call her in the evenings, suggesting 8:00 p.m. as a suitable time when he would be home and Claire's turtle patrols hadn't yet begun. Claire agreed, and they set the time for their nightly calls.

Time flew by, filled with swimming, lunch, and shared moments. But as the time came for Alekos to start his journey back to Nicosia, he retrieved his rucksack from his tent and bid farewell to everyone. After exchanging hugs and waves, he climbed the wooden steps with Claire close behind. He packed his rucksack into a small Mitsubishi Shogun, expressing his reluctance to leave. He hugged Claire warmly and kissed her, struggling to conceal his emotions.

"What have you done to this poor doctor's heart?" he teased gently before driving off towards Paphos, leaving Claire with a mix of emotions and the anticipation of their nightly calls.

After Alekos had left, Claire found herself surprised by how much she missed him and attempted to distract herself by taking long walks along the beaches. Maria caught up with her, and they sat together on the rocks at the end of the beach. Maria wasted no time in asking Claire about Alekos.

Claire explained that it was still early days and she wasn't sure how things would unfold, but she found Alekos to be a very kind person, so she thought it was worth taking a chance.

As they strolled back to their tent, Claire suddenly felt a strong urge to call Alekos. She retrieved her cell phone from her backpack and carefully made her way up the wooden steps in the dark. In the car park, she found a signal and dialed Alekos' number. After two rings, he answered, "Kalispera, good evening, is that my English Rose?"

"Kalispera Alekos, did you get home safely? I called because I was thinking about you," Claire replied.

"I'm delighted you did, Claire. I was thinking about you all the way home and am really looking forward to next weekend," Alekos confessed.

They exchanged a few more words before bidding each other goodnight with a virtual kiss. As Claire descended the steps back to the beach, she realized how happy and content she felt.

Despite missing a call from Alekos on Thursday evening, they managed to speak most evenings, and there was always so much to say. Claire couldn't shake off a sense of sadness, wondering why Alekos hadn't called, and imagining that he had changed his mind. However, she discovered the next day that his absence was due to his theater list running over on time, with several complicated operations keeping him occupied.

On Friday evening, when Alekos finally rang, he apologized for not calling and then extended an invitation to dinner the following evening. "I've checked with Nicos, and he can spare us for a few hours. I want to take you to a traditional taverna not too far from the turtle station where we can enjoy fresh fish sitting at a table overlooking the harbor," he suggested.

Claire was thrilled by the invitation and found herself unable to sleep that night. Their excitement was well-founded as they were kept busy the next day. Four new turtle nests were discovered, and Maria and Claire had the joy of witnessing one of the female turtles digging her nest in the light of the waning moon.

After the turtle had returned to the sea, Maria stood by the nest as Claire dashed to the hatchery to fetch one of the protective cages, which they both carefully placed over "their turtle nest".

Chapter 4
Moon Magic

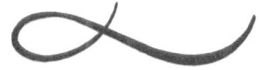

CLAIRE felt delighted to see Alekos descending the wooden steps to the beach the next morning. They all gathered around the wooden table, feeling a bit worn out after the busy night.

"Oh my goodness," laughed Alekos, "I think I need to brew some of our famous strong Cyprus coffees!" Everyone wholeheartedly agreed with him.

Feeling a bit tired, they spent much of the day lounging around the table, engaging in various discussions. Alekos frequently climbed up the sand dune to the car park to check his cell phone, as one of his patients was not recovering as well as expected.

By mid-afternoon, they all decided it was time to swim to the rock again in pursuit of eternal youth. When Claire asked Alekos if he was joining them, he regretfully declined, citing the need to regularly check in with the hospital from the car park.

As they swam, Kurt managed to complete the three circles around the rock in record time, boasting, "I'm going to look like I'm in my twenties when there are 100 candles on my birthday cake!"

While swimming back to the shore, Claire noticed someone on top of the sand dune—it was Alekos- wildly waving his arms and blowing her kisses. She couldn't help but laugh at his antics and accidently swallowed a mouthful of seawater in the process.

They all returned to the hut, dripping water in all directions, Alekos had prepared refreshing drinks for everyone. He then announced to the group that he and Claire would be heading out for dinner in St. George, resulting in loud applause and enthusiastic whistling from the others.

Claire and Maria volunteered to walk the beach after Nicos spotted some holidaymakers who had set up a sun umbrella in the sand. This was strictly prohibited due to the risk of damaging an undetected turtle nest. After politely explaining the issue to the holidaymakers and asking them to remove their umbrella, Claire and Maria set off for "their" rocks. Maria danced around her friend, bombarding her with questions and teasing Claire about her earlier proclamation that she didn't want any romance.

Maria asked Claire about her outfit for dinner, to which Claire replied, "Just shorts and a tee shirt, I didn't pack anything special." Maria's excitement was palpable when she realized her large Spanish shawl would complement Claire's outfit perfectly. She explained that her mother had suggested she take it in her backpack to protect her arms and shoulders from the sun.

An hour later, Claire emerged from the tent wearing the shawl tied around her waist and her hair styled in a French braid by Maria. Her friend embraced her and planted two large kisses on her cheeks before wishing her a happy evening. Feeling quite nervous, Claire climbed the wooden staircase to the car park.

Alekos was already by his car and rushed around to open the passenger door for Claire. Taking her hand, he gently kissed it and told her, "You look really special tonight - as beautiful as Aphrodite."

Twenty minutes later, they arrived at the harbor in St. George. Alekos opened the car door for Claire, took her hand, and they walked across the car park and up the steps to the taverna. Alekos had booked an outside table overlooking the harbor, which Claire found to be the perfect setting for their first date.

They ordered a fish Mezé, a popular Greek classic comprising numerous little 'taster' dishes to share. Alekos felt it was the perfect way for Claire to sample many different traditional Cypriot dishes. They were completely at ease in each other's company, discussing a variety of topics including the past week, hobbies, music, and the countries they would like to visit. Time flew by, and soon they found themselves walking back to the car.

As they reached the car door, Alekos pulled Claire close and kissed her gently. "Claire, I hope you enjoyed this evening as much as I have. I love spending time with you and being able to step inside your world, which is so different from mine. I would love to stay here another hour, but we had better not. I wouldn't like to cross Nicos, he could ban us from going out again!"

Back on the beach, they received news that a turtle had come ashore early to lay her eggs. Kurt had noticed the sound of flying sand not far from where they were eating their evening meal, and upon closer inspection, they found the turtle covering her nest with sand thrown backward using her powerful front flippers.

Her nest was not far from the rows of protected nests, so Nicos decided it would be best to leave it in place and just place a protective metal cage over the top of it.

Nicos had already divided the group for the beach patrols, and to Claire's disappointment, she and Alekos were in different groups. Claire giggled upon hearing that Alekos would be with Maria, as she was sure Maria would interrogate him with endless questions about the evening. Cypriots were definitely more direct in their questions than other nationalities, something Claire had noticed with Maria, Alekos, and Nicos.

The night passed uneventfully, with no more turtles coming ashore. Claire and Kurt were on patrol before Alekos and

Maria, so they had a few minutes to meet up, during which Alekos discreetly stroked Claire's arm.

Before they knew it, Sunday had arrived, and the day passed far too quickly for both Claire and Alekos. They took the chance to walk the beach mid-afternoon and spent time sitting on the far rocks. "Oh my goodness, Claire, why do I find leaving you so difficult?" Alekos pondered. "I start to miss you within five minutes of driving out of the car park. Shall I come back to Lara next weekend?"

Within an hour, they were both climbing up the wooden steps with heavy hearts. They shared a long, lovely kiss and cuddle before Alekos reluctantly climbed into his car. Through the open window, they shared a final goodbye kiss and agreed to speak later in the evening- each knowing how much they would miss each other.

Chapter 5
The Trials of Love

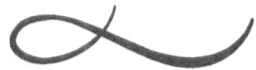

As the following weeks slipped by, Claire and Alekos settled into a workable routine. During the week, they focused on their respective roles, and at weekends, they cherished their time as part of the turtle team at Lara.

Alekos continued to excel in his work at the hospital, impressing Pavlos with his skill and dedication to his patients. Despite the long hours and demanding surgeries, Alekos remained committed to his profession.

Claire immersed herself in her work on the Turtle Project in Cyprus, relishing the opportunity to learn about marine turtles and to be able to contribute to conservation efforts. After 25 years of hard work, the project was showing promising results, with both species of turtles no longer experiencing a decline in numbers- although they remained endangered.

During quiet moments at the hut, Claire found herself wondering if her experience would have been even better with Alekos by her side. Their nightly phone calls became a lifeline, but Claire couldn't help but notice the exhaustion in Alekos' voice at times, a reminder of the demanding nature of his job.

One evening, as Claire returned from the car park, she found Nicos sitting in front of the hut. They began chatting, and Nicos expressed his observation of how happy and relaxed Alekos seemed when Claire was around. He thanked her for being a positive influence on his friend.

Nicos gently broached the topic of what would happen when Claire returned to England, prompting Claire to realize that she and Alekos hadn't discussed their future yet. She acknowledged Alekos' tendency to immerse himself in work and understood the importance of addressing their relationship when they next met in person.

Deciding that it wasn't a conversation to have over the phone, Claire resolved to discuss their future together face-to-face, recognizing the need for open communication and planning for what lay ahead.

As they walked along the beach, the water gently lapping at their feet, Claire broached the subject of her return to England with Alekos. His response was serious, indicating that he had already given it considerable thought.

"I've been thinking about it a lot, Claire," Alekos began. "I was wondering if you would like to come over to Cyprus when you can and stay in Nicosia? Maria and I discussed this last week because she really wants to stay in contact and see you regularly. She thought it would be great for you to stay with her so you can see me as much as possible."

He paused briefly before continuing, "It would be ideal if you could come over. I would be happy to pay for your flights because, you know, trying to get away can be difficult for me, and when I'm on call, it's absolutely impossible."

Claire agreed that Alekos' suggestion made sense and proposed that he might like to travel to England for Christmas. She described how London transformed into a winter wonderland in December, sharing her excitement about the festive season with him.

The atmosphere at the Lara Turtle Project was filled with anticipation as the last weekend in August approached, marking Claire's imminent departure the following Wednesday. However, there was also an air of celebration, as it coincided with Alekos' Name Day on the 30th of August. Nicos suggested they commemorate the occasion with a special meal.

Explaining the significance of Name Days in Cyprus, Nicos laughed as he observed their puzzled expressions. He clarified that in Cyprus, people often celebrate their Name Days rather than Birthdays, which are associated with saints' names, or they have been named after a grandparent- or often, or both! As Alexander's Feast Day fell on the 30th of August, it was a perfect opportunity to honor Alekos.

The volunteers at Lara enthusiastically came together to prepare a feast, not only to celebrate Alekos' Name Day but also to cherish their final moments together before parting ways. With most volunteers preparing to return home to resume their work or studies, the occasion held even more significance.

As they worked on the preparations, they also continued their regular patrols of the beaches, although the nesting season for turtles was coming to an end. While it was unlikely to encounter a female turtle laying her eggs at this time, they remained vigilant in their conservation efforts.

The combination of celebration and farewell created a bittersweet atmosphere, emphasizing the bonds forged during their time together at Lara and the memories they would carry with them as they parted ways.

Claire was eagerly anticipating Alekos' arrival at the beach on Saturday morning, so she was pleased to be patrolling the beach first thing in the morning with Maria, as they always had plenty to talk about.

The pair walked slowly along the beach, looking for the distinctive pattern in the sand made by the turtles' front flippers as they hauled themselves towards the water, but there was nothing.

They sat on the rocks at the end and looked back towards the tents.

"I'm really going to miss being here," said Claire with a sigh. "It's been amazing to be part of such a special project," she added. "I can't believe that the female turtles we've seen have been coming ashore every two weeks to lay their eggs, and it's highly likely that they were born here at Lara, so they instinctively know to return here."

"It's certainly been great fun," agreed Maria. "I'm so pleased to have met you and hope that our friendship lasts for many years," she said as she impulsively hugged her friend. "You've had the best time of all, finding love here too. Please come and stay with me whenever you can. I like to think you will—to see me, as well as Alekos," she added with a big grin. "Have you talked about the long-term future with him? What do you both plan?"

Claire shook her head and said that it was a subject she must address in the next two days. They stood up and started walking along the beach. Maria slipped her arm into Claire's and asked nervously, "You do want to stay in contact, don't you? You will send me messages often." Claire gave her friend a huge hug and promised her that she would.

As they reached the four rows of metal cages protecting the turtle nests, they stopped to closely check each for any movement that could indicate that the eggs were starting to hatch. The incubation period is 49-60 days, so in addition to patrolling the beaches, the volunteers were taking care to check the nests every few hours too.

They were just checking the final cage when Claire noticed a familiar figure walking down the wooden steps and quickly told Maria that she would see her at the hut, as she raced across the sand to meet Alekos. She was delighted to see him—and so were the other volunteers, who had all grown to like this gentle, caring doctor.

The rest of the day was spent walking the beaches, swimming to the rocks, and sitting outside the hut chatting. Claire and Alekos volunteered to check the other beaches, which gave them the opportunity to simply stand and hold each other tenderly.

The second time they were walking along the first beach, Claire plucked up the courage to ask Alekos about the months ahead. He turned to look at Claire and held her gently by the shoulders. "I am glad you have asked me," Alekos said. "The subject has been weighing very heavily on my mind. We have had such a wonderful time since we met that being so far apart is going to be awful—but we can make it work, we really can."

His eyes filled with tears, and he said the last words as though he was trying to convince himself. "I have been thinking of several solutions. You have one more year of study to complete, and I think we will have to try to see each other as often as we can until you graduate. I have already applied for leave to come to England for Christmas, and I would love you to come to Cyprus for the Orthodox Easter as it is so special. Hopefully, you can fly over for a few weekends too. It is going to be a very difficult time for us both, but I think we can make it work - 'S'agapo poli' – 'I love you very much'."

They held each other very close for a few moments, and then Alekos kissed Claire as she closed her eyes and brushed his lips with hers, replying, "Yes, we will make it work."

They returned to the main beach to find the large table in front of the hut filled with a tempting array of international dishes that they had all made. Nikos embraced his friend and wished him 'Chronia polla' - 'many happy returns' for his Name Day. 'I think that everyone has conjured up a magnificent feast bearing in mind we only have a two-ring cooker,' he added, laughing.

Everyone thoroughly enjoyed the evening, although Claire admitted afterwards that she had mixed emotions and a head filled with ideas about the forthcoming year and how hard it would be.

Claire stood outside her university and sighed. The weeks spent working as a volunteer on the Lara Turtle Project already seemed like a dream. Leaving Alekos and Cyprus had been incredibly difficult.

Alekos had not been able to get time off from the hospital, so Nicos and Maria had taken Claire to Paphos Airport for her flight home. They had laughed and chattered all the way, but Claire was finding it hard to be cheerful.

They both gave Claire a big hug. Nicos thanked Claire for all her hard work and said that there would definitely be a volunteer's place on the project the following year. Maria became tearful as Claire announced it was time for her to go through to Departures. Turning around to give them both a farewell wave was incredibly difficult, and her longing to be with Alekos was almost overwhelming.

Getting back into the university routine took time, and even seeing all her friends again didn't ease the missing she felt for Alekos. The hours passed far too slowly, and several times she had caught herself staring out of the window and not hearing anything the lecturer had said.

She looked forward to speaking to Alekos every evening. They would spend ages chatting through their days before telling each other "S'agapo para poli" - "I love you very much".

After she had been home ten days, a white envelope was waiting for her when she returned to her flat share. The envelope was covered in colorful Cypriot stamps. Claire eagerly opened the envelope to find a cute card and a confirmation sheet with flight details to Larnaca for her October break.

Claire held the envelope and paper tightly to her heart as she smiled to herself in relief– this was not just a holiday romance.

Chapter 6
Strengthening the Bond of Love

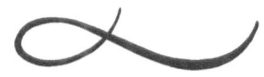

THE WEEKS luckily sped by for Claire as she was so excited about flying to Cyprus to see Alekos in October. She had to keep herself well-grounded as she was now in her final year with her final exams looming like thunder clouds on the horizon. The evening telephone conversations with Alekos were great – a real lifesaver - but just not enough; she longed to feel his arms wrapped around her again.

Soon all the waiting was over and she was walking swiftly to the departure gate to board the flight for Larnaca. Alekos had chosen her a seat on the left side of the cabin as he thought she may be able to see Lara Bay as the aircraft started its descent as it approached Cyprus.

Alekos was standing in Arrivals right by the barrier, and his face was completely transformed by a huge smile as he spotted Claire. He rushed forwards and gently steered her away from the barrier so that he could share the magic of holding her again. The drive to Nicosia flashed by as they both had so much to say to each other. Maria was nervously waiting for them at her apartment where she had prepared them a special meal for them all to enjoy.

Claire was delighted to see her friend again, and the evening passed by far too quickly; suddenly it was time for Alekos to leave as he had work early the next morning.

Like Claire, Maria was on holiday from university so intended to show her new friend all the treasures of the city each morning. This included the little workshops where craftsmen created beautiful copper pots, painted ceramic plates, stitched elegant tailored suits and made stylish leather jackets.

Most afternoons, Maria and Claire studied, but on one, Maria took her to meet her parents and enjoy lunch with them. Claire spent the evenings with Alekos, and he took her to different restaurants including a Lebanese one near the old city walls - which Claire had particularly enjoyed.

The four days flashed by, and soon they were sharing their final evening together. Claire looked across the table at Alekos and timidly raised the subject of Christmas and whether he would be able to get over to the England. She realized that her heart was pounding in case he said 'no'. Alekos smiled and said that he would certainly be able to and then carefully produced an envelope from his jacket pocket. He removed the typed letter inside and handed it to Claire to read.

Claire noticed it was a formal letter from the world-famous King's College Hospital in London. She read the letter twice to ensure that she had not made a mistake and let out a little squeal of delight! Immediately after Christmas, Alekos was going to be working at the hospital for two weeks so he could have in-depth training on an exciting new surgical procedure.

Claire was delighted as they would be able to see each other over the Christmas holiday and the weekend when Alekos was working at the hospital. Knowing this somehow lessened the pain of her leaving Cyprus.

As quickly as she had arrived in Cyprus, she was now on her way back to Larnaca Airport. As her check-in was an early one, Alekos had been able to arrange to drive her to the airport. There had been hugs and tears from Maria as she left Nicosia and she had proclaimed that she wanted her English friend to stay in Cyprus forever.

Checking in for the flight felt horrible as Claire so wanted to just turn around and leave with Alekos. It took all her courage to remain cheerful and stoic. Alekos tenderly pulled her close to him and kissed her on her eyelashes before brushing his lips against hers.

They walked in different directions as Alekos returned to the car park and Claire headed for Security and then Passport Control. As the aircraft took off, Claire studied the island's coastline and spotted the large sweeping bay of Lara. Moments later, the aircraft pierced through the fluffy clouds, and the last few days became a happy memory.

Christmas passed just as quickly for Claire. Having such a fun time with Alekos actually made the missing harder, she decided. Alekos stayed in London with Claire's sister and friends, who made him very welcome. He loved all the British Christmas traditions, which seemed so different from the Cypriot ones. Alekos was amazed by the light decorations in the main shopping streets and had loved the winter wonderland in Hyde Park. The ice skating had proved challenging to them both and there had been much laughter. They had enjoyed sitting snuggled up together with a mug of warm mulled wine and doing some Christmas shopping.

After Christmas, Alekos started his time at King's College and loved every minute of it. He felt that he would burst with all the fascinating new ideas he had gleaned from the neurologists and couldn't wait to tell Pavlos all that he had learned.

Claire and Alekos had managed to see each other a couple of times during the week, which they had both enjoyed. Claire's parents had treated them to seats at one of the shows in London, which Alekos had enjoyed but had declared was 'very, very British!' During the weekend, they bought bus tickets for the open-topped bus in London, so that they could jump on and off at all the different famous sights.

In a twinkling of an eye, it was time for Alekos to return to Cyprus. Claire's father offered to take him to the airport and waited discreetly in the car park so that Claire could walk with Alekos into Departures and say goodbye without worrying about what her father was thinking!

The months between Christmas and Easter passed agonizingly slowly because there had been no chance for Claire to go to Cyprus as the pressure was definitely on now at university. The Greek Orthodox Easter rarely coincides with Easter in the England, so Claire was only able to spend a few days in Nicosia. It was enough, though, to enjoy time with Alekos, to meet his family, and to experience all the traditions of the Greek Orthodox Easter.

On their final day together, Alekos said that they would be meeting up with Nicos for lunch. It was great to see Nicos again, and Claire teased him that he was unrecognizable as he was dressed in a suit rather than shorts and a t-shirt! The three of them chatted happily together about the turtle project, days at Lara, and the forthcoming season. Nicos asked Claire whether she would like to be a volunteer for the summer.

"Much as I would love to," said Claire, "a great deal depends on whether I am successful in getting a job as I am in my final year. I have only just started to apply," she explained with a mock terrified face!

"Aaah," said Nikos, "I was going to ask you about your plans. You see, there will be a vacancy in the Department of Fisheries here in Nicosia in October, but you would need to get a good grade for your degree - and to learn Greek," he added with a big grin! "With Alekos and Maria as your tutors, I think this could be possible," said Nikos.

"Wow," said Alekos, "What do you think, Claire?"

Claire was sitting looking quite shocked as she had not expected a job offer as well as a tasty lunch! She asked if the men minded if she went outside to ring her parents.

A few minutes later, she returned looking relaxed and very happy. Her parents had thought it was all wonderful, and her father had said that he would love regular holidays in Cyprus. They felt that the job offer was great as it meant she could concentrate on her exams without worrying about the future. They really liked Alekos and could see how happy he made her, so the most important point of all is that she could be with him and be able to support him in his work.

Her father had declared it was a 'win-win situation' and that he would be cracking open the excellent bottle of Cypriot wine that Alekos had given them at Christmas!

With just a few months until she moved to Cyprus, Claire worked incredibly hard to ensure she finished her time at university on a high. She spent any free time learning Greek online – which she said was the greatest challenge of all.

Claire moved to Cyprus in late June and two boxes with all her possessions were sent by her parents to arrive once she and Maria were back in Maria's flat after their time at Lara. While she was at the turtle station, she heard that she had passed her degree well and it had been a good excuse for a celebration meal on the beach with Alekos and the other volunteers the following weekend.

It was during one of the weekends on the beach as they watched a female turtle return to the sea that Alekos asked Claire if she would marry him.

Amidst the laughter and kisses he said that he had already asked Claire's father for permission to do so, and her father said yes, joking that he should give him a whole case of wine as a thank you.

In front of both their proud families, the couple were formally engaged at a church in October and preparations began for a traditional Greek wedding the following May.

A May wedding meant there was nothing to disrupt the ever-important turtles' nesting season. And they were both sure that with their love for each other, there was nothing that could ever disrupt their happiness.

Epilogue
5 Years Later

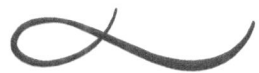

CLAIRE sat on the balcony of the Claire sat on the balcony of the apartment in Nicosia that she and Alekos had moved into after their honeymoon in Paris. She loved to watch the sun sink in the sky. Alekos had telephoned to say that an emergency operation had been added to his list and he would be late coming home.

She had been busy herself and was quite happy to relax for a little while.

She sighed as she thought about how five years had sped by in a happy blur of work, families, and magical times with Alekos. Claire patted her stomach gently and smiled. She was really looking forward to being a mother and Alekos was so excited about the baby.

She would be leaving work to go on maternity leave in two short weeks as their baby was due on their wedding anniversary – 14 May. Claire would return to work leaving her baby to be cared for by Alekos' mother who was unbelievably excited at the prospect.

For now, she was happy to just relax and enjoy the moment, remembering how it had all started on a very special beach in Cyprus...

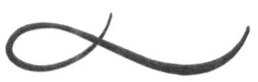

Other Books from Seniorality

To find your next Seniorality book visit:

www.amazon.com/author/seniorality

Where you will find:

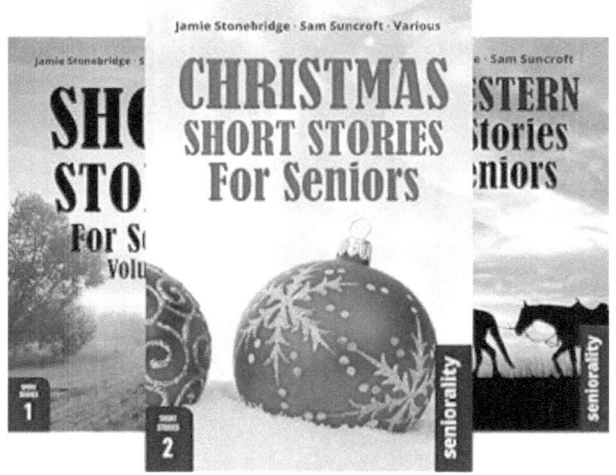

Short Stories

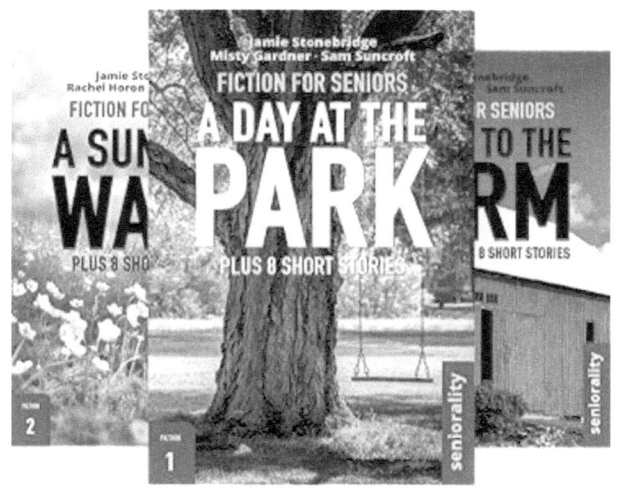

[Fiction for Seniors](#)

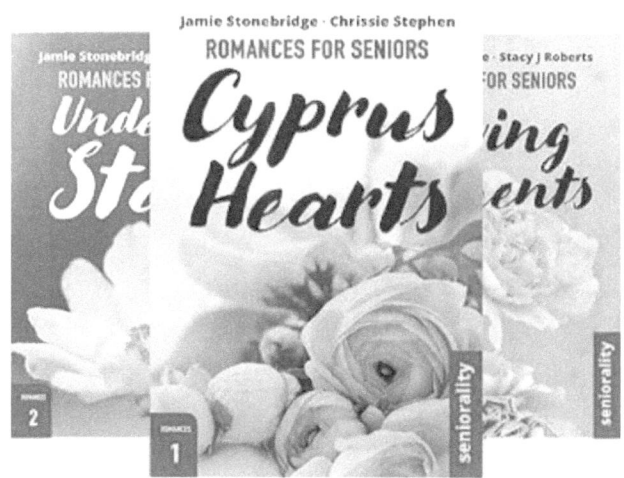

[Romances for Seniors](#)

Find these and many more books
by searching on Amazon for 'seniorality'
or visit: **www.amazon.com/author/seniorality**

Thank You

If you enjoyed this book or found it useful, we'd be very grateful if you'd post a short review on Amazon. Your support really does make a difference and helps other people discover this book.

We read all the reviews personally so we can get your feedback to make ours books even better or get ideas for future books.

Thank you and have a wonderful day!

www.ingramcontent.com/pod-product-compliance
Lightning Source LLC
Chambersburg PA
CBHW020441220526
45464CB00002B/808